Table of Contents

All about Blood Pressure 3
Who Can Develop High Blood Pressure? 6
Are You at Risk for High Blood Pressure? 9
Why Do We Develop High Blood Pressure? 11
What Can Raise Your Blood Pressure? 14
What Should You Know If You Have High BP 17
Children and Blood Pressure 20
Your Child's Blood Pressure 22
Monitoring Your BP at Home 24
Finding the Right BP Home Monitor...26
Benefits of Early BP Monitoring 28
Understanding Your BP 31
Understanding Your BP Numbers...34
High Blood Pressure 101 37
Tips for Controlling Your Blood Pressure...................................40
Preventing High Blood Pressure 42
Diet and Food Affect Your Blood Pressure 45
Lowering Your Blood Pressure 48
Options for Dealing with High BP 50
How Does Exercise Help? 52
Taking Control of Your BP...55
BP Control = Health Control 57
All about BP Medication 60

When To Use BP Medication 63

Remembering To Take BP Medication 66

All about Blood Pressure

What is blood pressure? Blood pressure is the force of your blood against your artery walls. When you have your blood pressure checked the reading has two numbers; one on top and one on bottom.

The top number is your systolic pressure. This is the force of your blood in your arteries when your heart beats. The bottom number is your diastolic pressure. This is the force of your blood in your arteries when your heart relaxes in-between beats.

Normal blood pressure would be a reading of 120/80 or lower. High blood pressure would be a reading of 140/90 or higher. If you have high blood pressure you are at a greater risk of a stroke or heart and kidney disease.

Many things can cause high blood pressure including physical inactivity, tobacco and alcohol use, stress and your diet. These are only a few things. Certain medical conditions and medications can also cause high blood pressure.

High blood pressure can cause your body to have certain effects. For instance it can cause a stroke. The high pressure can cause a weakened blood vessel to break causing it to bleed into the brain; thus leaving you with a stroke.

High blood pressure can also sometimes cause your blood vessels in your eyes to bleed or burst. If this happens your vision will be blurred or impaired and might even result in blindness. Another reason it is best to keep control on your blood pressure.

Along with a stroke or kidney disease high blood pressure can also cause a heart attack. Your arteries are what bring blood carrying oxygen to your heart muscle. If your heart is not getting enough oxygen you will experience chest pain. If the blood flow is blocked as well you will experience a heart attack.

Congestive Heart Failure is very common among people with high blood pressure. This is a very serious condition where your heart cannot pump enough blood to supply the needs of your body. It is never too late to start taking control of your health starting with your blood pressure.

Anyone can develop high blood pressure, even children. It is more common for African Americans to develop it. Many Americans will develop high blood pressure as they age but that doesn't mean it is healthy.

Obesity plays a role in high blood pressure. If you are overweight you are at a higher risk of having high blood pressure as well as a stroke or heart disease. Try to lose at least ten pounds and this will help lower your blood pressure significantly.

Eating a healthy diet is a great way to lower or control your blood pressure. Limit your intake of salt and sodium and introduce more fresh fruits and vegetables into your diet. Once you establish your healthy diet you will have less worry of developing high blood pressure.

You should always have your blood pressure checked at your regular doctor visits. If you have high blood pressure and are concerned you can easily monitor from home. If you do this you want to have your doctor look at your home monitoring device to help ensure it is effective and you are operating it correctly.

Keep track of your blood pressure readings so you can see what is helping and what isn't. Sometimes regular lifestyle changes alone won't help as much as they would combined with blood pressure medication. Your doctor will be able to tell you what the best option for your needs would be.

Who Can Develop High Blood Pressure?

Are you battling high blood pressure? Do you feel like you are the only one? You shouldn't feel that way because millions of Americans have high blood pressure. Only a certain percentage of them actually know it.

When you see your doctor you have your blood pressure checked. Some people think this is irrelevant because they say they will never have high blood pressure. Probably one of the reasons so many people do not even know they have it. They think for whatever reason it won't happen to them.

While it can be frustrating to monitor your blood pressure, there are things you can do to help lower it or keep it under control. Exercise is a great way to lower and control your blood pressure.

Close to one in three American adults have high blood pressure. While high blood pressure is very common among Americans, African Americans tend to get it while they are young and more often than white Americans.

Whatever your age or gender or ethnicity, you can easily prevent and control your high blood pressure. There are simple ways like exercising and even simple lifestyle changes to do this.

If you are overweight you are at a greater risk of high blood pressure. The higher your blood pressure is the higher your risk of stroke or heart disease is. Exercising can help you lose weight and also lower your blood pressure.

Eating healthy is also a great way to control blood pressure. Eating the right fruits and vegetables and foods altogether is proven very beneficial. Using less salt and sodium makes a huge difference and also drinking very minimal alcohol.

Tobacco also increases blood pressure, so if you smoke or use any kind of tobacco product, consider limiting yourself if not quitting altogether. You may find it easier to slowly wean yourself from it.

Stresses plays a major factor in blood pressure and let's admit it, everyone gets stressed at one time or another. If you find yourself dealing with a large amount of stress, you should try some relaxation techniques. Consider meditation, or whatever it is that relaxes you. Do this when needed and you will see a significant improvement in the way you feel.

Did you know the cause of ninety to ninety-five percent of high blood pressure is unknown? Luckily high blood pressure can be easily detected and controlled with multiple options.

Another interesting statistic shows that people with less educational and even income levels usually have higher blood pressure. Do you wonder why this? Maybe a lot of that is stress!

It doesn't really matter who can develop high blood pressure, it's controlling it that matters. If you are battling high blood pressure or just want to take necessary precautions to help prevent from getting it, see your doctor. Ask any and all questions and they can help you find a great effective way to lower or control your blood pressure.

Remember to exercise and try to eat healthier. These overall will work wonders and you can thank yourself in the end when your body does.

Are You at Risk for High Blood Pressure?

Do you know what the risks are of high blood pressure? How do you know if you are at risk? There are many different causes for high blood pressure. In this article you will find out if you are at risk and how you can help prevent and control your high blood pressure.

Your blood pressure is high if it is over 120/80, which is the normal level of blood pressure. There are many everyday lifestyle habits that raise your pressure that you might not be aware of. One of those is being overweight. If you are overweight you are at a greater risk of developing high blood pressure.

Try to start a healthy diet or start exercising. Even losing a measly ten pounds can help you drastically and keep your blood pressure normal. Physical inactivity is also another lifestyle habit that causes many Americans to develop high blood pressure.

If you are not very physically active, consider starting to be. You can easily adapt exercise to your everyday routine; you just have to plan it out. Try to do at least thirty minutes of exercise a day. This will help lower or control your blood pressure.

Many people are not concerned with what they eat, yet they want to be healthy. These two do not go together. If you want to stay healthy, you have to watch what you eat. Having unhealthy eating habits can cause high blood pressure as well. Try to eat less salt or sodium and more vegetables and fruits.

Using tobacco products is a great risk for developing high blood pressure. Smoking is a very common habit among the world and many of these people might have high blood pressure and not even know it. There are many ways to help rid the habit of nicotine or use of any tobacco product.

Everyone is stressed at some point during their lives. You might be stressed every day or just once in a while. Whatever the case may be, you can still develop high blood pressure through stress. If you find yourself stressed more often than not, consider some relaxation techniques. Meditation is a great way to start. If this doesn't work, consider something different.

Drinking alcohol also causes high blood pressure. Do you drink quite a bit? More than two drinks for a man and more than one for a woman can raise their blood pressure. If you drink more than this, consider cutting back. Once again, if you are addicted to drinking, or smoking, you can find many ways to help you quit.

These are very common lifestyle habits that cause high blood pressure. If you are at risk for high blood pressure or already have it, consider purchasing a home blood pressure monitoring device. This can help ensure that whatever habits you are changing or modifying are working.

Sometimes this change is not enough. You might have to use medication or incorporate medication with your exercise routine, etc. The best way to know this is to visit your doctor. Ask any and all questions you might be concerned about. They will happy to assist you in helping you have a healthier and active lifestyle.

Why Do We Develop High Blood Pressure?

You might wonder why you and everyone else develop high blood pressure. While you might develop it you can easily lower or control it. The best way to prevent developing it is to keep a close eye on it from the beginning.

Older adults may be more prone to developing high blood pressure but if you start at a young age you can prevent it easier. There are a few things you want to watch for that cause high blood pressure. This is why we develop high blood pressure because we are not aware of what is causing it.

Weight plays a major role in developing high blood pressure. Overweight people are more likely to develop high blood pressure but do not be discouraged. Losing as little as ten pounds can help your blood pressure significantly.

Once you lose a measly ten pounds just imagine how much easier it will be to lose even more. A great way to keep losing and maintain a healthy weight is by a healthy diet. Your diet factors in to developing high blood pressure as well.

High amounts of salt and sodium intake can cause high blood pressure. Try to limit your meals on salt and opt for other seasonings instead. There is a wide variety of seasonings available so you are sure to find something you really like.

Also try to incorporate fresh fruits and vegetables into your diet. Eating more of these will help your blood pressure not to mention you will feel healthier as well.

Do you use tobacco or drink large amounts of alcohol? If so, this could be why you have developed high blood pressure. Both of these can raise your blood pressure so if possible try to quit or at least cut back on your use and consumption. This will significantly help lower or maintain a normal level of blood pressure.

African Americans are more prone to develop high blood pressure. It starts at an early age and can be more severe. African Americans also have a higher death rate from kidney disease and stroke than white Americans. Even so, you can still treat high blood pressure effectively.

Do you exercise regularly? If not you might be at risk for developing high blood pressure than those that do regular exercise. Luckily you can easily fix this by doing physical activity for at least thirty minutes a day. You might say, "I don't have thirty minutes a day to set aside." While you may not have thirty minutes all at once to set aside, you could probably find it easier to set aside ten minutes at a time.

If you find yourself stressed very easily over anything and everything you could easily develop high blood pressure. Yes, stress is a factor of high blood pressure. Stress is very common for many people but easily treatable. Is there something you enjoy doing that relaxes you?

Consider picking up a hobby that you find relaxing and lets you de-stress. Do this whenever you feel stressed to the max and do it often. Keeping your stress level low will help keep your blood pressure low as well.

Last but not least, certain medications can cause you to develop high blood pressure. Are you on medications? You might consider talking with your doctor about their side effects and if they cause high blood pressure. Every time you start a new medication you want to ask your doctor about this.

It is never too late to take better care of your health so consider starting today. Keeping control of your blood pressure will help lower your risk of a stroke or heart and kidney disease. Talk with your doctor about any concerns or ask any questions you might have.

What Can Raise Your Blood Pressure?

Are you concerned about what might increase your blood pressure? There are quite a few things that can factor in to raising your blood pressure. Luckily you can fix many of these with a few lifestyle changes.

If you do not watch your blood pressure frequently, you might not even be aware that you have it. It can creep up on you or just increase over the years. It all depends on many different factors.

If you are overweight you are at an increased risk of developing high blood pressure. You might already know this and you might not. If this is the case for you, consult your doctor and see what he might recommend for you. Losing at least ten pounds can significantly lower your blood pressure.

An unhealthy diet or lack of physical activity or exercise can also put you at risk for high blood pressure. Try to exercise at least thirty minutes a day even if you have to space the time out. Eating less salt and more vegetables and fruits can help lower your blood pressure as well. Try to incorporate this into your present diet and you will see the results rather quickly.

Stress plays a huge factor in high blood pressure and unfortunately everyone is stressed at some point in their lives. If you deal with a high amount of stress, consider relaxation techniques. Do whatever you can that you know will calm you down and help relieve stress.

Using tobacco and alcohol raise your blood pressure. If you use either of these consider quitting. If you are unable to quit right away, limit your consumption of alcohol and use of tobacco. There are many over the counter and prescription products to help rid yourself of these habits. Talk with your doctor of any concerns you might have.

Medical conditions also factor into high blood pressure along with your lifestyle. Kidney disease can result in high blood pressure as well as cause it. Sleeping disorders that interrupt your breathing during sleep will also raise your blood pressure. Talking with your doctor about your condition could benefit your disorder along with your blood pressure.

Certain medications and drugs can also raise your blood pressure. Certain types of anti-depressants will do this as well as certain cold medicines. Be aware of oral contraceptives, nasal decongestants, anorexia drugs and steroids. These can possibly raise your blood pressure as well so talk with your doctor before taking any of them if you are concerned.

While you can control most of the factors that raise your blood pressure there are some you cannot. For instance your race; African Americans are more prone to high blood pressure, people over fifty-five are at a higher risk, and your family history can play a role in your blood pressure as well. While you cannot control these factors you can easily try to help decrease your risk. Watch your diet, exercise, lifestyle habits, etc. Over time this may be very beneficial to you.

High blood pressure can cause strokes and even heart and kidney diseases. Leading a healthier life style can help you live longer and enjoy your time in a healthy state. Talk with your doctor about any questions or concerns you may have concerning your blood pressure. It is never too late to take control.

What Should You Know If You Have High BP

If you are battling high blood pressure there are some things you will want to know. First thing you want to understand is what the numbers mean. Your blood pressure will read with a top and bottom number. The top is your systolic pressure and the bottom number is your diastolic pressure.

Normal blood pressure is 120/80 so if your blood pressure reads 130/90 you are at risk for developing high blood pressure. This reading is called prehypertension which is basically a stage before developing high blood pressure.

By having your blood pressure checked and monitored often you can easily lower it where it needs to be. The best way to do this is by maintaining or adopting a healthier lifestyle. Have you always had normal blood pressure until recently?

If this is the case, consider what you have recently started doing different that may have caused it to rise. Did you change your diet? Have you been exercising less? Maybe you are on a medication; some medications can cause your blood pressure to rise.

If you do have high blood pressure you can easily monitor it at home if you choose. If you do this you still want to keep your regular doctor visits. You can share your own results and you can both see what is and isn't working for you.

If you are on other medications consult your doctor. Chances are one of these could be raising your blood pressure and you want to take control as soon as possible. If your blood pressure gets too high without proper treatment you are at more risk of having a stroke or heart and kidney diseases.

If you have recently changed your diet you should talk to your doctor, especially if your blood pressure has risen since then. Lots of salt and sodium can cause high blood pressure and not enough fresh fruits and vegetables. If this is the case, try to limit your salt intake and get more vegetables in your diet.

Also physical inactivity can be a cause for high blood pressure. Have you recently stopped doing regular every day physical activity? If so, consider starting again. You might have stopped because of an inevitable reason; broken bone, etc. If this is the case talk with your physician, together you can find a way to still get a little bit of physical activity in your daily routine.

You also want to cut off or limit your use of tobacco and alcohol consumption. Many people do not realize these cause high blood pressure. There are many over the counter medicines and even doctor prescribed medicines to help you quit smoking. There are also many different resources to help you quit drinking.

If your doctor prescribes blood pressure medicine for you, you want to be sure and remember to take it. Some people are bad at remembering to take medication. There are many different ways you can help yourself remember.

You take the risk of a stroke or heart disease by not taking your blood pressure medication. This should be reason enough to take your medicine, but sometimes people just forget. While it sounds like reason enough, if you are not used to taking daily medication it is rather easy to forget.

If you have certain questions or concerns talk with your doctor. They will gladly answer any questions you have and do their best to get your blood pressure at a normal rate again.

Children and Blood Pressure

Did you know that even babies can develop high blood pressure? Many might think of this as uncommon but it isn't. When babies have high blood pressure it is usually because they are premature or have kidney or heart problems. When an older child has high blood pressure it is usually a result of their family history.

As you might have noticed today, there is an increase in obesity in children. This also increases their blood pressure putting them at health risks. A great way to prevent this is to have your child's blood pressure checked often as they grow older.

More ways to help are watching your child's diet and making sure they get plenty of exercise. Some kids are not as active today what with the video games and all. Try to get your child involved in regular activities from the start. It will benefit their health as well as their self-esteem later down the road.

Just like adults, you can easily help control your child's blood pressure. Watch their diet. Be sure they are getting the right nutrition and limit their salt intake. Get them eating vegetables and fresh fruits. While many children do not like vegetables, there are many ways to overcome this. You can spice up a recipe that involves vegetables.

Physical activity is the key to any healthy lifestyle. Getting your child involved in physical activity when young will help ensure they stay active and healthy as they age. Involve them in sports of their choosing and take walks with them. You can both benefit from this.

If your family has a history of high blood pressure, be sure your child gets routine check-ups. This will help ensure they do not develop high blood pressure and if they do, you can start controlling it. Remember stress can raise blood pressure and while some kids shouldn't be stressed, they are.

Children deal with stress just like adults, just in different ways. Talk with your child and stay active in their life and what goes on. You want them to have a happy healthy life and you can help them achieve that goal.

If you are unable to control your child's blood pressure through their diet and exercise, you might have to turn to medication. Talk with your doctor and let them know what you have already tried. Sometimes this is not enough alone, but with medication, can help control it.

Try to exercise with your child every day. Exercising alone sometimes is harder for children and adults alike. You can get involved with your child this way and it will benefit you both.

Talk with your teenager about smoking and drinking. These both cause high blood pressure and once they know the risks they are less likely to try them. Do not think your child is invisible from developing any health problems along with high blood pressure.

Remember that blood pressure increases with age until you are around fifty. If you get a head start on watching yours and your child's at an early age, you will both benefit very well in the end.

Your Child's Blood Pressure

You may not realize that your child can develop high blood pressure. While it may not always be the case, it isn't uncommon by any means. You can take control of your child's blood pressure while they are young and help them live a healthier life.

Obesity is the main cause for children to have high blood pressure. Researchers say that obesity is increasing every year in children. This might be due to video games and other activities that require no physical activity. You can easily prevent this luckily.

Start by getting your child active. You can exercise with them every day for thirty minutes. Take a walk, ride your bikes, go swimming. Whatever physical activity you choose will benefit you both.

By involving your child in physical activities at a young age, you are increasing their chance of staying active as they get older. Limit their video game time, etc. You don't want to banish all 'fun' things but they should know that sports and physical activities can be fun as well.

Also watching your child's diet and eating habits can be beneficial in controlling their blood pressure as well as your own. By starting a diet for the entire family, your child will not feel 'cornered' or 'picked-on'. The entire family will be doing it so it will not be just for them.

When starting a new diet for controlling your blood pressure there are many things you will want to do.

• Limit your sodium and salt intake. Substitute salt for other seasonings.

• Introduce more fresh fruits and vegetables. By early introduction of fruits and vegetables in your child's diet, you can ensure they will continue to eat these as they age.

• Monitor Fiber Intake - For children one to three they should have 19 grams of fiber a day. For children four to eight they should have 25 grams of fiber daily. For female children nine to thirteen they should have 26 grams of fiber and for males 31 grams. For females fourteen to eighteen they should have 29 grams and for males 38 grams of fiber.

• You as an adult also want to consume 14 grams of fiber per thousand calories consumed. You can easily read the nutrition labels to make sure you are getting the recommended amount.

You also want to watch the amount of fat intake. This of course will cause obesity along with physical inactivity; which both of these will raise blood pressure. Try to have balanced healthy meals and send your child to school with a balanced lunch. You can find things they will like that has the appropriate nutrition.

Children should have the opportunity to be children and eat some junk food as well. Choose a day or time that your child can eat something like this. After all, this is probably the only time they'll be able to enjoy eating something like that. Let them be a kid but also have a healthier lifestyle. You will both be thankful and grateful further down the road.

Monitoring Your BP at Home

If you are concerned about your blood pressure you should consider monitoring it from home. You still want to keep your regular doctor visits but this will help ensure you are making the right lifestyle choices. There is nothing more frustrating than changing your entire lifestyle for your blood pressure only for it to show no change. While this can sometimes happen, you might just need to add medication.

If you decide to monitor your blood pressure at home you want to keep a record. By doing this you can see what is working and what isn't in lowering or maintaining your blood pressure.

When monitoring your blood pressure you have choices of the equipment to use. You can use an aneroid monitor that has a dial gauge and uses a pointer to read. You can also use a digital monitor with the option of a manual or automatic cuff. With a digital monitor your reading will flash on the screen.

Some people might suggest using a finger or wrist monitor but these have been proven less effective. They are not as accurate, more movement sensitive and more costly as well.

When choosing your monitor you want to choose one that has the right cuff size for you. If you are unsure of what size to get, ask your doctor. If the cuff size is wrong your reading will be wrong, therefore you receive no benefit in the end.

If you want to be sure you are operating the blood pressure monitor right take it to your doctor. They can show you how to use it correctly. Using it the right way will ensure you get the right readings.

There are certain things you should to before checking your blood pressure. You do not want to drink or use any caffeine, alcohol or any tobacco products thirty minutes prior to checking. You want to be sure you use the restroom first as well. Relax and don't talk for at least three to five minutes prior to taking a reading.

Make sure you are completely comfortable. Do not cross your legs or arms and keep your back straight. When you strap the cuff on, you want to be sure your arm is at the same level of your heart. Rest it on a table or solid surface. Be sure the cuff is snugly fit around your arm but still has room for a finger. The bottom of the cuff should be an inch from the crease of your elbow.

Understand what your numbers mean before monitoring your blood pressure from home. Normal blood pressure would be a reading of 120/80 or less. High blood pressure would be 160/100 or higher. Anything in between these readings would mean prehypertension and this means you are on the way to developing high blood pressure.

You want to avoid this at all costs if possible and if you find your numbers increasing consult your doctor. Together you can find an effective way of helping you decrease your blood pressure. You might even have to consider blood pressure medication.

Finding the Right BP Home Monitor

If you are checking your blood pressure from home you have the choice of choosing your own monitor. You can use either an aneroid monitor or a digital one. There are advantages and disadvantages to both.

An aneroid monitor has a dial gauge and your blood pressure is read by a pointer. You inflate the cuff by hand using a rubber bulb. With a digital monitor you can choose a manual cuff or an automatic one. You can read your blood pressure reading on a screen digitally as well. You want to choose the one you are more comfortable using.

An aneroid monitor is very portable. The cuff that comes with this monitor also has a stethoscope built into it. The aneroid blood pressure monitors range cheaper in price compared to the digital ones. A down side to this monitor is that it may be too hard for some people to hear as well as too hard to squeeze the bulb.

Digital monitors are the more popular blood pressure monitoring devices because they are automatic. Unlike the pointer on an aneroid device, the digital device shows your numbers on a screen. This makes it a lot easier to read. You can even purchase a digital monitor that comes with a paper print out feature. This would make it easier to keep a record of your blood pressure readings.

The digital monitor has a gauge as well as a stethoscope. With the digital monitor it has an error code which can be very beneficial and automatic deflation of the cuff. With a digital monitor you have to use batteries and depending on the model you may have to use your left arm. You can purchase a digital monitor anywhere from thirty dollars to ninety and higher.

You want to choose a blood pressure monitoring device with a cuff that is the right size for you. The right cuff size will ensure correct blood pressure readings. Ask your doctor if you are unsure of what size you need. Be sure you can easily read and operate the device.

If money plays a factor in your decision choose a device that fits your needs as well as your budget. When it comes to your health you have to decide if you can really put a price on it. While you do not want to spend an unreasonable amount of money on something like this, you still might have to splurge a little extra.

Look around and see what your options are. You might know someone that has a home blood pressure monitor. If so, ask them what they might recommend. They might recommend whatever device they are using now or tell you to steer clear of it.

You want to choose one that is easy for you to use and read. Be sure you can understand how to operate it as well. The less confusing it is to use, the more beneficial it will be. Imagine how much better you are going to feel once you gain control of your blood pressure. It will be much simpler by monitoring from home as well as having regular check-ups at your doctor visits. Lower blood pressure lessens your risks of a stroke or heart and kidney disease. This alone should make you feel much better.

Benefits of Early BP Monitoring

Did you know that your blood pressure increases as you age? By taking control of your blood pressure at an early age you can have the benefit of a longer healthy life. In this article you will find ways to monitor your blood pressure and the benefits that come with it.

If you are unable to have regular check-ups at your doctor's office, you can purchase a blood pressure monitoring device. If you have a history of having high blood pressure a monitor is a great way to keep an eye on it.

Since blood pressure increases with age it is best to start monitoring it as early as possible. Many young people do not worry about things like this, but if your family history involves high blood pressure, it is best to start now.

The first thing when monitoring your blood pressure is to know what makes it increase. The following are just a few things that can cause it to increase.

Smoking and Alcohol

Tobacco use and alcohol can drastically increase your blood pressure. The best way to prevent this is to sustain from using tobacco or drinking alcohol. If you do not desire to do this, you can try limiting your use of tobacco and alcohol consumption. If you have tried quitting either before there are many available resources to help aid you in completely quitting.

Overweight

Being overweight will also drastically increase your blood pressure. If you can try to lose at least ten pounds this will help significantly.

Physical Inactivity

Do you exercise regularly? If not, you might want to start doing so. Exercise can help lower your blood pressure. Try doing at least thirty minutes of physical activity every day. If you cannot set aside thirty minutes at one time, try doing ten minutes at a time. As long as you get thirty minutes a day you will see results.

Stress

Yes, stress can raise your blood pressure. If you find yourself stressed every day, consider doing something to help you relax and de-stress. Meditation or a similar relaxation technique will do wonders with dealing with stress.

Your Diet

If you have an unhealthy diet, this could be the cause of your blood pressure increase. Try to limit your salt intake and introduce more fresh fruits and vegetables in your diet. Read nutrition labels and try to eat less fat, etc.

Sleeping Disorders

Sleeping disorders can raise your blood pressure because your breathing is interrupted while you're sleeping. You can fix this by talking with your doctor about medication to help you sleep.

There are many available medicines that have proven to be effective in helping sleeping disorders.

Over-the-counter drugs, substances and supplements

Some over the counter medicines and other supplements can trigger high blood pressure; specifically antidepressants, cold medicines, oral contraceptives and nasal decongestants. If you are worried about a certain medication you are currently taking, consult your doctor. Ask any and all questions you may have concerning your blood pressure.

By watching all this you can stay away from the risks of high blood pressure including stroke and heart or kidney disease. It is never too late to start taking care of your health.

Understanding Your BP

What is blood pressure? Blood pressure is the force of your blood against the walls of your arteries. Blood pressure consists of two number; a top and bottom number. The top number is the systolic pressure. The bottom number is the diastolic pressure.

Systolic blood pressure is the force of blood in your arteries as your heart beats. If your systolic number is higher than one hundred and forty you have high blood pressure. Even if your diastolic number is not high you can still have 'isolated systolic hypertension.' This means only your systolic number is high.

This is more common for older Americans. This pressure usually increases with age whereas diastolic pressure decreases after fifty-five. You might not know if you have isolated systolic hypertension so ask your doctor if you are concerned.

Diastolic blood pressure is the force of blood in your arteries when your heart relaxes between beats. For younger people this is a very important number. The higher this pressure is the more you are at risk. This blood pressure lowers as you get older and your systolic increases. Therefore diastolic is more important in younger people and systolic in older.

Normal blood pressure is less than one hundred and twenty over less than eighty. If your pressure is between the normal numbers and one hundred and thirty-nine over eighty-nine, you have what is called prehypertension. This puts you at risk to develop high blood pressure in the future but it easily preventable.

Hypertension is a name for high blood pressure. Having high blood pressure puts you at risk for heart disease or even strokes. High blood pressure makes your heart work harder than it should and can lead to blindness, kidney disease and even congestive heart failure.

According to statistics high blood pressure killed over fifty-four thousand people in 2004. Statistics also show that twenty-eight percent of people have high blood pressure and aren't even aware of it. Are you one of them?

You should be aware of the risks of high blood pressure so you can avoid them as best as you can. High blood pressure is a risk for stroke and heart disease. While some risks can be altered or fixed, some cannot. For instance if you use tobacco or are overweight you are at risk for high blood pressure.

You can easily fix this by trying to quit using tobacco and watching your diet to help lose weight. If you have trouble doing either of these on your own, consult your physician. They may be able to prescribe you something or give you useful information to help.

High blood pressure can affect certain parts of your body as well. You might suffer from a stroke. This happens because the high blood pressure can break a weak blood vessel leaving it to bleed into the brain. Also if you have a blood clot blocking a narrow artery, you can also experience a stroke.

Sometimes impaired vision or blindness can occur from high blood pressure. It might eventually cause your blood vessels in your eye to bleed or burst leaving you with blurred or impaired vision.

Your arteries harden as you age, even more so for those in your heart, brain and kidneys. These harder arteries are associated with high blood pressure. When this happens your kidneys and heart have to work harder.

If you have any questions or concerns about your blood pressure ask your doctor. They can answer any questions you might have and find a solution if you do in fact have high blood pressure or might be prone to it. It's never too late to take care of your body, including your blood pressure.

Understanding Your BP Numbers

Are you concerned about your blood pressure? If so, you can easily start monitoring it in your own time in your own home. You still want to have it checked regularly by your doctor. The best way to monitor your blood pressure is by understanding the numbers first.

There is a top and bottom number for your blood pressure reading. The top number is your systolic pressure. Systolic pressure is the force of blood in your arteries as your heart is beating.

The bottom number is your diastolic pressure. Diastolic pressure is the force of blood in your arteries as your heart relaxes between each beat.

There are four different categories your blood pressure reading can fall under. The first is a normal blood pressure reading. Normal blood pressure is when your systolic pressure is below 120 and your diastolic pressure is below 80. This would read 120/80. You can keep this blood pressure number by maintaining a healthy lifestyle.

The second category is 'prehypertension.' This is where your systolic pressure reads 120-139. Your diastolic pressure would be between 80 and 89. This would read as 121/81 or 139/89. If you have prehypertension just maintain a healthy lifestyle to keep your blood pressure from increasing.

The third category is called Stage 1 hypertension. This is where your systolic pressure is between 140 and 159 and your diastolic pressure is between 90 and 99. If you have a reading like this, try to adopt a healthier lifestyle. If you cannot lower your blood pressure on your own, talk with your doctor about medication.

The fourth category is called Stage 2 hypertension. This is where your systolic pressure is 160 or higher and your diastolic pressure is 100 or higher. If you have this high of blood pressure consider adapting a healthier lifestyle and talk with your doctor about taking medication to help lower it.

While you can easily watch your diet and weight and get plenty of exercise to help maintain or lower your blood pressure, that may not be enough. Blood pressure medication might be prescribed by your doctor and you might even have to take two.

If this happens be sure you tell your doctor of any other medication you might be taking. Some medications including antidepressants, cold medicines, nasal decongestants and even oral contraceptives can raise your blood pressure.

Like usual, talk with your doctor about any concerns you might have and if you have any questions about your blood pressure. There are many available ways to treat high blood pressure and you want to be sure to find the right option best suited for you.

By taking control of your blood pressure you can take control of your health and have a longer healthier life. If you smoke, try to quit, try to limit your alcohol consumption and eat lots of fruit and vegetables.

If you have a dog, take a walk with them every day. Get yourself at least thirty minutes of physical activity. You will be thankful you did when you realize how much better you feel.

High Blood Pressure 101

Knowing about your body can be very beneficial to your health as you age. Knowing about your blood pressure can help prevent strokes, heart disease and kidney disease. In this article you will find everything you should know about your blood pressure.

Anyone can have high blood pressure. It doesn't matter your age, race, ethnicity or gender. Many people suffer from high blood pressure and have a higher risk of strokes and heart diseases than those with regular blood pressure.

What is high blood pressure?

High blood pressure is the force of blood against the walls of your arteries. Your blood pressure is always rising and falling throughout the day and if it rises and stays that way over time, you have high blood pressure.

High blood pressure is usually referred to as hypertension. When you have high blood pressure it puts more pressure on the heart, making it work harder than usual. This is why you end up at risk for strokes or heart disease.

What is the normal blood pressure level?

The normal blood pressure level is less than 120 over 80 or less. The first number is your systolic pressure and the second number is your diastolic pressure. Your numbers are read 120 over 80, etc. If your pressure is 140 over 90 or higher you have high blood pressure.

What is systolic blood pressure?

This is the force of blood in your arteries when your heart is beating.

What is diastolic blood pressure?

This is the force of blood in your arteries when your heart is relaxing.

What are the risk factors of high blood pressure?

The most common risks of high blood pressure are stroke and heart disease. There are a few other risk factors that can be modified and some that cannot be. The following are some risks:

- Tobacco

- Physical Inactivity

- Diabetes

- Abnormal Cholesterol

- Being overweight

Who can get high blood pressure?

Unfortunately anyone can get high blood pressure but it is more common among African Americans. Nearly one in three American adults has high blood pressure. African Americans also have a much higher death rate from kidney disease and stroke than white Americans. Even so, with treatment you can help lower your blood pressure.

How can I lower my blood pressure?

Fortunately there are many different ways of helping to lower your blood pressure. Exercise is a great way to lower it. Doing physical activity will make your heart stronger over time. If you have a stronger heart it can pump blood easier lessening your risks of stroke and kidney diseases. It is never too late to start exercising!

If you are concerned about your blood pressure consult your physician. Ask any and all questions you might have and find the best way for you to lower it. If all regular ways fail, consider medication. Talk with your doctor about your health and lifestyle so he can choose the best medicine for you. If you want to live a healthy life, taking control of your blood pressure is very important.

Tips for Controlling Your Blood Pressure

Do you have high blood pressure or at risk to develop high blood pressure? If so do not be discouraged, there are ways of controlling and lowering your blood pressure without medication. Simple lifestyle habits are the most common causes for high blood pressure and easily helped.

Keep in mind that sometimes everything you try may not work. You might have to have the help of medication along with your healthier lifestyle. Talk with your doctor first. They will be able to assist you with the best option for your lifestyle.

The first thing you can do is achieve a healthy weight if you aren't already. Being overweight is a great risk for developing high blood pressure. You can avoid this by watching your diet and reaching your healthy weight.

If you are unsure of what your healthy weight should be, you should talk to your doctor. You can even find a site online that lets you calculate your BMI (body mass index) and this will tell you what your healthy weight is.

Exercising should be a normal part of your lifestyle. Not everyone enjoys exercising and even if you are one of those people, you can still add it to your everyday routine. Only thirty minutes a day of exercise will greatly decrease your risk of high blood pressure.

If you cannot set aside thirty minutes at one time, do ten minutes at a time. This is just as effective and you can get thirty minutes in your day quicker and easier than you thought. You can walk or run or whatever you like.

Your diet plays a major role in your blood pressure levels as well. A high intake of salt and sodium can greatly increase your risks. Try to limit yourself on salt and sodium intake and have your doctor advise you on the recommended amount according to your blood pressure levels.

Using herbs and spices in place of salt is a great way to reduce your salt intake. When you go out to eat somewhere, suggest 'no salt' or ask if they add salt so you know if you should or not. Many people consume tons more salt than they really should and do not even know it.

Stress plays a big role in high blood pressure and unfortunately many people suffer from stress. The best way to help your own is by finding a relaxation technique that works best for you. Try meditating, or something that has always relaxed you before. Let the stress of the day leave you and enjoy your stress free time. Take as long as you want to do this.

While trying to change your lifestyle habits, try to keep a record as well. Grab a notebook or journal and write down what you did and check your blood pressure often. Note if it is making a difference or staying the same.

If lifestyle changes do not help as much as you would like, you might consider talking with your doctor about taking medication. Sometimes lifestyle changes alone aren't as effective unless used with medication. Talk with your doctor about any concerns you might have and they can help decide what is best for you.

Preventing High Blood Pressure

If you are battling high blood pressure there are many ways to lower it and prevent yourself from developing it again. The best way to start is without medication if you can help it by making some lifestyle changes.

Do you smoke? If so, this can raise your blood pressure. Try to cut back if not quit altogether. There are many aids that can help you quit smoking. Do you drink quite a bit of alcohol? This will also raise your blood pressure so try to cut back to a drink or two a day.

Do you consider yourself physically active on a daily basis? Getting at least thirty minutes of exercise a day has been proven to lower and maintain a healthy blood pressure level. Do ten minute intervals if you cannot set aside thirty minutes all at one time.

Start a healthier diet. Did you know salt increases your blood pressure dramatically? Limit your intake of salt or substitute it for other seasonings. There are so many different seasonings available you should have no trouble finding one you really like.

Add plenty of vegetables and fresh fruits into your diet. This will also help lower and control your blood pressure. Try to stay away from fatty foods as well.

If you are overweight this could have a major impact on your blood pressure. Losing as little as ten pounds can significantly reduce your blood pressure. Once you lose ten pounds you will see how easily you can lose more and you will notice how much better and healthier you feel. Not to mention your blood pressure levels will decrease.

Do you have a stressful job or life? Try to do away with as much stress as you possibly can. If you cannot avoid all the causes of stress in your life find something that helps you relax and de-stress. Meditation might work wonders for you.

There are certain things you cannot avoid that have an effect on high blood pressure. Your race: African Americans are at a higher risk. If you are older than fifty-five you are at risk as well and unfortunately you cannot make yourself younger.

If you have a family history with high blood pressure, you want to start early prevention. Knowing about your family history will help in cases like this. Even if you do not have high blood pressure now you have the risk of eventually developing it, but that doesn't have to happen. Early prevention can keep your blood pressure down.

Stay away from drugs and painkillers if possible as they can cause high blood pressure. Some prescription medications can cause high blood pressure such as: nasal decongestants, anorexia drugs, steroids, antidepressants, oral contraceptives and cold medicines.

If you are taking any of these and are having problems with your blood pressure levels, be sure your doctor is aware you are taking them.

Having high blood pressure can put you at a higher risk of stroke and heart and kidney disease so preventing this can benefit your health immensely. Talk with your doctor of any questions you might have or concerns. No question is silly and it is never too early to start taking better care of your health starting with your blood pressure.

Diet and Food Affect Your Blood Pressure

Are you aware that what you eat can affect your blood pressure? Watching your diet can be very beneficial to keeping your blood pressure normal. Even if you have never had a problem with high blood pressure, taking necessary precautions can be beneficial.

You could try a Vegetarian diet. In this diet you will get many of the following:

• Calcium

• Magnesium

• Vitamin A & C

• Potassium

• Complex Carbohydrates

• Polyunsaturated Fat

• Fiber

All of these can have a great influence on your blood pressure.

Sugar can increase your blood pressure, especially the common table sugar sucrose. Try to limit your intake of this. A diet high in fiber has been proven effective in lowering blood pressure. Along with lowering your blood pressure this diet will also help you reduce your cholesterol levels and even promote weight loss.

Eating plenty of fruits and vegetables is very important as well. Any diet that includes consuming fruits, vegetables, low-fat dairy foods and is low in total fat, cholesterol and saturated fat has proven to be effective in lowering blood pressure.

Many people use more salt than they are aware of. Maybe because some of us are just used to automatically salting our food unaware if it was salted when being cooked. (If eating out) Reducing your salt intake will also help lower your blood pressure.

A diet high in potassium and low in sodium reduces your blood pressure rise by reducing the effect of adrenaline. If you reduce your sodium intake you must also increase your potassium intake.

There are some vegetables and spices that help control your blood pressure. Many of these are very common vegetables and spices so you may be helping your blood pressure and not even know it.

Onions' essential oil is very beneficial. If you have two to three tablespoons of this essential onion oil a day, it could help reduce your systolic levels. Tomatoes are also a beneficiary to controlling blood pressure. They are high in GABA, a compound that helps lower your blood pressure.

Broccoli contains several blood pressure reducing ingredients. Carrots also have many compounds that do the same. Introducing these vegetables to your diet will do wonders for your blood pressure. Even if you don't suffer from high blood pressure, it's best to keep it at a safe level and take the extra precautions to get there.

Garlic and celery are also great to add to your diet. Garlic is good for the heart which you've probably been told before. Eating just one clove of garlic a day has been proven to be beneficial.

Whatever diet you choose or whatever foods you try to limit, remember you are doing it for your health. Many people learn to enjoy healthier foods as they get older. If you have any questions or concerns about your blood pressure get with your doctor. They will be happy to assist you and answer any questions you might have. Taking care of your health is very important and will make you feel much better.

Lowering Your Blood Pressure

Do you have high blood pressure? Maybe you want to prevent getting high blood pressure, no matter what the case is, there are everyday things you can do. What you eat, how much you exercise, even your habits can affect your blood pressure.

If you see your doctor regularly you more than likely have your blood pressure checked every time. This is a necessary procedure to monitor your pressure and be sure you don't have high blood pressure. There are different reasons one has high blood pressure and different things you can do to help lower it.

If you have high blood pressure it damages your blood vessels increasing your risk for stroke or heart and kidney diseases. In other words, having high blood pressure is very harmful to your health and you want to treat it right away.

Making lifestyle changes is the first way to go when you want to lower your blood pressure. If doing these simple changes does not help and you have to use medication, continue doing the changes along with the medication. The lifestyle changes alone may just not be enough and added with medication could help significantly.

If you use any tobacco of any kind, stop your use or decrease it significantly. Nicotine makes your blood vessels constrict resulting in a faster heart beat. This faster heart beat raises your blood pressure. You can easily find products that help quit smoking or help quit the use of other tobacco products.

If you are overweight you are at a high risk of high blood pressure. Start a diet program and start eating healthier. Exercising regularly is very beneficial to lowering your blood pressure. Plan an exercise routine and track your progress. This will show you what is working and what is not.

Eat plenty of fruit and veggies and try a low fat diet. Try to stay clear of sodium, alcohol and caffeine or at least limit your intake. Sodium isn't harmful to everyone's blood pressure but until you know for sure, it is better to take precaution.

Alcohol can cause high blood pressure in some people as well. Try to only drink one or two alcoholic beverages a day. If you know this is increasing your blood pressure, try to quit altogether. Your health might be at risk.

Stress can sometimes affect your blood pressure. Stress is very common and there are millions of ways to help reduce stress. Try some relaxing techniques first and if none of these work talk to your doctor. They may have some better suggestions.

If all else fails you may have to turn to medication. There are many types of medicine to help you lower your blood pressure. You may end up taking this medicine for the rest of your life but if it helps keep you healthy, it is worth it.

If you are still unsure of how to handle your blood pressure talking with your doctor is the best solution. Tell them of your concerns or ask them any questions you might have. No question is stupid when it comes to your health. You could even do some research online and find out many things about blood pressure. You are not the only one curious about taking care of your health. Take the necessary steps to live a long healthy life.

Options for Dealing with High BP

If you are battling high blood pressure do not be discouraged. Did you know that as many as seventy two million people in the U.S. 20 and older have high blood pressure? Twenty eight percent of these do not even know they have it.

Some people do not worry about their blood pressure until they get older. While this might make sense to an extent, it is never too early to monitor your blood pressure. If you have a family history of high blood pressure, you want to start right away.

How many people wait until they are diagnosed with something before attempting to prevent it or cure it? Too many. By taking control of your blood pressure today you can prevent a stroke or developing heart or kidney disease later in life.

When you are young you might be more active than when you get older. Try to stay active and if you aren't, get active. All it takes is thirty minutes a day of physical activity or exercise to control your blood pressure and better your health.

Eat healthy foods. Try to stay away from salty and fatty foods. Salt increases your blood pressure and fatty foods might cause weight gain, which causes high blood pressure as well. Try to eat more vegetables and fresh fruits. You might find you like more than you thought you would.

Stress can cause high blood pressure but there are so many ways to de-stress. Do you have a favorite hobby that has no stress? If so, try to do this every time you feel yourself overwhelmed or stressed out. You will be surprised at the wonders it can do.

If you take medications talk with your doctor to make sure they aren't affecting your blood pressure. Certain medications can raise your blood pressure. Antidepressants, cold medicines, oral contraceptives, steroids, even nasal decongestants might be affecting your blood pressure without your knowledge.

If you are unsure of your family history, check it out. If you have a family history of high blood pressure chances are you will end up with high blood pressure as well. If you are aware of this early on, you can start monitoring and controlling your blood pressure before it gets a chance to become high.

There are many different kinds of blood pressure medications if you are unable to see results with regular lifestyle changes. Sometimes these medications are needed along with a regular healthy diet and exercise to be more effective.

The best thing you can do is talk with your doctor. They can suggest something that will help you control your blood pressure and even prescribe you some medication. If you start medication, be sure you tell them of any other medicine you are taking as well.

You want to be in charge of your health and not wait until something happens to take that control. When it comes to your health you can never be too late so start as early as you can. You are never alone when it comes to dealing with your blood pressure and other health issues.

How Does Exercise Help?

Do you want to take control of your blood pressure? If so, exercise may be the key for you to do just that. Many people may not realize exercise can help you control your blood pressure. Fortunately, it is all rather simple.

As you probably know, you are more prone to high blood pressure as you age. Unfortunately, we all age and this cannot be helped. But controlling your blood pressure can be helped.

By exercising you can prevent risks of high blood pressure which can cause stroke and kidney disease. If you already have high blood pressure, exercising can help you get it under control.

As you exercise your heart gets stronger. When your heart is stronger it can pump more blood more easily causing less pressure on your arteries. While exercise may not work for everyone you can easily lower your blood pressure by around ten millimeters.

Even if you do not have high blood pressure, you can take these precautions to prevent from getting it. Along with controlling your blood pressure you can lose weight or maintain your desired weight which also affects your blood pressure.

Overweight people are prone to having high blood pressure and an increased risk of stroke or kidney or heart diseases. If this is you, get moving and start exercising! This doesn't mean you have to overdo yourself, take it slow at first and work your way up. You will start feeling better as you continue a regular routine.

It is suggested to do at least thirty minutes of exercise a day if possible. Thirty minutes can be hard to do for some people, mainly because they can't find the time. If this is the case, you can do short bursts of exercise. You could exercise for ten minutes at a time throughout the day. At the end of the day you've done thirty minutes.

Like with starting any exercise routine, you will want to talk with your doctor first. There are certain things you will have to have your doctor's okay for. If you are a man over forty or a woman over fifty it might be better to talk with your doctor first.

Smoking increases blood pressure as well as makes it hard for some people to exercise. Being overweight has an effect on everything and you definitely want to consult your doctor before starting an exercise program.

Having a chronic health condition or high cholesterol and even high blood pressure can put you at risk when exercising. Be sure to talk to your doctor first. If you do not visit the doctor regularly, do so now. It is better to know exactly what health you are in before doing any strenuous activity or even exercising.

Always warm up before starting an exercise routine. Begin slowly so you can slowly build the intensity. Be sure to continuously breathe throughout your routine. Holding your breath can cause your blood pressure to increase and the key of exercising to help control or lower your blood pressure.

If you experience any discomforts or pain while exercising notify your doctor immediately. It is better to take full precaution even if it ends up being something little. Once you start your exercise program, you want to track your progress.

A great way to do this is if you can't see your doctor regularly; purchase a home blood pressure monitoring device. You want to check your pressure before you begin and when you are finished. You want to make sure it's working and how much it's working.

By exercising you are lowering your chances of getting high blood pressure and if you already have it, you are helping to control it. This means you are lessening your risks of strokes or heart diseases. It is never too late to start, no matter your age, gender, or ethnicity. Talk with your doctor today about an exercise program that is right for you. Your body will thank you in the end.

Taking Control of Your BP

Do you have problems controlling your blood pressure? Is it like a roller coaster ride? You do not have to worry any more. In this article you will find out how to take control of your blood pressure and have the healthy lifestyle you want.

As you may know there are many things that can cause your blood pressure to increase and many ways to decrease it and keep it that way. Your lifestyle will play a major role in this and even your race, age and family history.

You cannot change your race or age or history but you can still gain control of your blood pressure. African Americans are more prone to developing high blood pressure as well as people over fifty-five. You definitely cannot make yourself younger or change your color but that doesn't mean you cannot control your pressure.

Having a healthy diet will have a major effect on your blood pressure. If you like eating salty foods this might be hard for you, but well worth it. Having high blood pressure can lead to heart and kidney disease as well as a stroke.

Try cutting back on any salt and sodium in your diet. Your doctor will probably recommend a certain serving amount or intake amount of sodium for your diet. Also try to eat more vegetables and fresh fruit. These will make you feel a lot better along with decreasing your blood pressure.

Are you very active physical wise? Physical inactivity can play a huge role in high blood pressure. If you do not exercise regularly try to get in the habit. Thirty minutes a day is recommended but you can space the time out if needed. Do ten minutes here and there and before you know it, you've done thirty minutes of physical activity.

Do you smoke or drink? These will raise your blood pressure as well. Quitting either of these habits can be tough, but there are many helpful resources out there to help you. If you know you cannot quit right away, try limiting your consumption and use. Set a certain amount to smoke and drink a day.

Slowly lower the amount and before you know it you will be ready to quit. Try doing this along with medication or something that helps you quit. Doing small things like not being around anyone that smokes or drinks can help immensely. Also try replacing these habits with something else. If you get the urge to smoke or drink start doing something else you enjoy.

Do you have a stressful job or just a stressful lifestyle in general? Stress can increase your blood pressure. You want to find a way to de-stress and relax. Is there a certain hobby that does this for you? You might also try some relaxation techniques such as meditating. Do these as often as you need to help keep the stress away.

If you are still concerned about your blood pressure talk with your doctor. By telling them any concerns and asking any questions you might have, they can better help you find the best way to control your blood pressure. Sometimes medication works better than anything else.

BP Control = Health Control

Do you realize by taking control of your blood pressure you can also take control of your health? Who doesn't want to have a healthy and long life? Taking care of your body can help ensure you get to endure that long healthy lifestyle you want.

You should be receiving regular blood pressure checks at your regular doctor visits. If you want to check it more often than you go to the doctor, you can purchase a home device that lets you monitor your blood pressure. There are different kinds to choose from.

Two of those are the aneroid and digital monitor. There are ups and downs to both monitors so you want to choose which one is best for you. The aneroid monitor uses a pointer to let you read your blood pressure. The digital monitor displays your reading on a screen which makes it easier to read.

The aneroid monitor is cheaper than the digital but requires more work from you. Check them out and even discuss with your doctor which one might be better for you. Once you purchase it, have your doctor show you how to effectively use it.

Among taking your own blood pressure readings, you can double check your lifestyle habits. Are you on a healthy diet? Eating healthy will help keep your blood pressure low and normal. Cut back on salt and sodium if you can't get rid of it altogether. Opt for seasonings instead.

Introduce more vegetables and fresh fruits into your diet. Once you become used to eating certain foods, it will be easier to do it every day. Before you know it you will be in the habit of eating healthy foods and won't think twice before doing so.

If you use tobacco or drink excessive amounts of alcohol try to cut back or refrain completely. These will raise your blood pressure putting you at more risk for a stroke or heart disease.

If you cannot quit these on your own there are plenty of resources and medications to help you. Talk with your doctor about the best way to go about quitting.

Would you consider yourself at a healthy weight or overweight? Overweight people are more prone to developing high blood pressure and if this is your case, try to lose at least ten pounds. You should see results in your blood pressure as well as the way you feel.

If you are not already regularly physically active, try to do at least thirty minutes of physical activity or exercise every day. This will help lower your blood pressure as well as make you feel a whole lot better.

If you find yourself lacking motivation to do some of these things, talk with a friend or relative that could buddy up with you. Having someone to exercise with or take on a challenge such as quitting smoking or drinking can help drastically.

Having high blood pressure puts your health at risk and that alone should be motivation but to some it isn't. Do not be discouraged, there are many ways to help lower your blood pressure.

If these lifestyle changes do not help, consider medication. There are many different kinds of blood pressure medications and sometimes they need to be combined with a healthy lifestyle to work more effectively.

If you have questions or concerns about your blood pressure talk with your doctor. Let them know what you want and they can help find the way that is best for you to control or maintain your blood pressure letting you control your health as well.

All about BP Medication

Have you tried changing your lifestyle to help your blood pressure only to find it isn't helping very much? Sometimes lifestyle changes alone aren't as effective as when combined with blood pressure medication.

There are many different kinds of blood pressure medications out there today. Usually two different medications are used rather than one alone. Here are some of the main blood pressure medications:

- Alpha-Blockers: This medicine reduces nerve impulses to your blood vessels allowing easier flowing of the blood making your blood pressure decrease.

- Alpha-Beta-Blockers: These work just like the alpha-blockers but also slow your heart beat. This means less blood pumps through your vessels making your blood pressure decrease.

- Nervous System Inhibitors: This medication relaxes your blood vessels by controlling the nerve impulses making your vessels wider and decreasing blood pressure.

- Beta-Blockers: These reduce your nerve impulses to your heart and blood vessels, making your heart beat decrease while dropping your blood pressure.

- Diuretics: These are also known as 'water pills,' a very common medication. These diuretics work in your kidney, flushing out all excess sodium along with water from your body.

- Vasodilators: These open your blood vessels directly by relaxing the muscle in your vessel walls which then causes your blood pressure to decrease.

- ACE Inhibitors: ACE stands for 'Angiotensin converting enzyme.' These inhibitors prevent a hormone called angiotensin II from forming, which will usually cause your blood vessels to narrow. They help the vessels relax which makes your blood pressure decrease.

- Angiotensin Antagonists: These block your blood vessels from angiotensin II. When blocked these vessels can widen letting your blood pressure decrease.

- Calcium Channel Blockers: These keep any calcium from entering your heart's muscle cells and your blood vessels causing your blood pressure to decrease.

An alternate to taking any medication if possible is watching a few lifestyle habits. For instance a healthy diet can help control your blood pressure. Substitute salt for other seasonings and add lots of fresh fruits and vegetables to your diet.

Get at least thirty minutes of physical activity or exercise a day. That doesn't mean you have to exercise thirty minutes all at once. Ten minutes here and there is just as effective.

Try to keep your stress level at a minimum. High stress can increase your blood pressure so find something that relaxes you and helps you de-stress. Do this whenever you find yourself stressed out beyond your means.

Try to cut back on tobacco use and alcohol consumption. Quitting altogether is more beneficial but isn't always easy. Remember there are many resources and products available to help you quit either of these habits.

Sometimes these lifestyle changes will not work alone. Your doctor might prescribe you a blood pressure medication if not two. Just talk with your doctor to find out what would be better for you and your blood pressure. Ask any and all questions and if you are taking other medications tell your doctor. Certain medications including oral contraceptives and cold medicines can increase your blood pressure.

When To Use BP Medication

If you are concerned about your blood pressure there are different types of medication you can take to help control or lower your pressure. You might try some lifestyle changes first before opting for medicine. Remember that sometimes medicine is the only way you might be able to lower it. Different lifestyle changes do not always work on their own.

First you might consider your diet. Do you consider yourself a healthy eater? Do you think you have a pretty healthy diet? Your diet could be affecting your blood pressure. High amounts of salt and sodium intake can raise your blood pressure. Try to limit your salt intake and eat more fresh fruits and vegetables.

If you love salt, consider substituting it with a different seasoning. There are so many different kinds of seasonings available you can easily find something to your liking.

Are you physically active on a regular basis? Physical inactivity can play a part in high blood pressure as well. If you can try to get at least thirty minutes a day of physical exercise you can help lower or control your blood pressure.

If you cannot set aside a full thirty minutes do ten or five minute intervals. As long as you get thirty minutes total for the day you are helping your blood pressure. This could mean taking a walk, doing an exercise video, riding a bike, etc. Whatever physical activity you enjoy the most will benefit your health and blood pressure.

Do you use tobacco or drink high amounts of alcohol? This can dangerously increase your blood pressure. Try to limit your tobacco use or alcohol consumption. If you can, quit them altogether. This is not always easy for some but do not feel discouraged.

There are many products to help you quit both habits and just focus on knowing you will feel healthier and you will be controlling your blood pressure too. If you have high blood pressure you are at risk for a stroke or heart and kidney disease. This alone should be motivation enough to get healthier.

While some of these lifestyle changes alone may not help you, it is always worth giving it a shot. If all else fails talk to your doctor about starting a blood pressure medication. Just remember to keep trying the lifestyle changes along with taking your medication. Doing both can significantly help your blood pressure.

There are many different types of blood pressure medications and sometimes two will work better than one alone. If you do not like taking medicine this can be rather hard to accept but know it will benefit your health in the end.

A few types of blood pressure medications are beta-blockers, diuretics, vasodilators, alpha-blockers, alpha-beta-blockers and nervous system inhibitors. These are only some of the many available blood pressure medications.

Before taking any blood pressure medications or starting any new diet you want to consult your doctor. They might be able to help you choose something that will help your blood pressure without drastic changes or measures. Ask them any questions or concerns you have. This is your health you are discussing and you want to know everything.

If he suggests a medication ask him what it does what the side effects are and if it will interact with any other drugs you might be taking, prescription or non-prescription. You can never be too careful and avoiding a stroke or heart disease is very important if you can help it.

Remembering To Take BP Medication

Are you currently taking medicine for your blood pressure? Do you take other medication as well? Remembering to take any medicine can be a hassle to some people especially if you have to take more than one at a time. Here are a few things that might help you remember because it is very important you do not forget to take your blood pressure medication.

Some people purchase little pill boxes that help you organize your pills. You can purchase pill boxes that have one for every day of the week. You put all the pills you need to take into each box for each day. You can purchase these almost anywhere and they do come in handy for those that are forgetful.

If you take medicine regularly you might try keeping it on your bathroom sink. When you finish getting ready or even just brushing your teeth, you can take your medicine. Have your blood pressure medicine and any other medication that you have to take right there. This is a great easy reminder.

Get into a routine. Taking your blood pressure pills at the same time every day will eventually get you in the habit and you won't forget. If you have to take your medicine with food you could always take them every day with your lunch. Getting in the habit of this is a great way to never forget your blood pressure pills again.

There are many people that put notes everywhere to remind them to do something. Taking your blood pressure medicine is no different. Put up a note on your fridge or on your computer at work. Every other day or every week change the color of the